KEEP FIT WITH
DRINK

THE ALCOROBIC WAY
TO BUILD A
A BETTER BODY

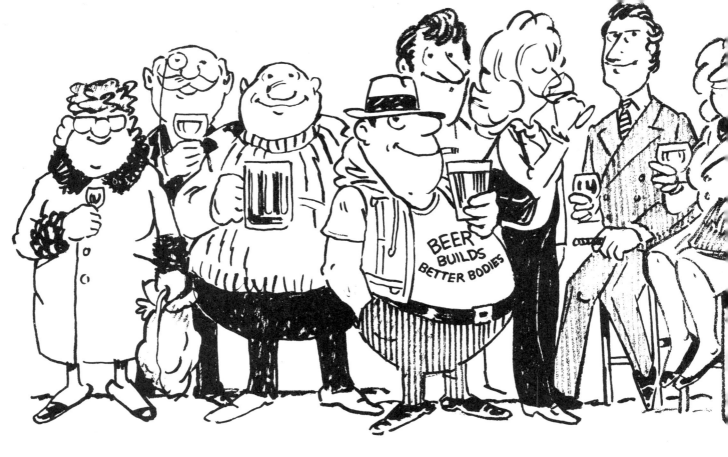

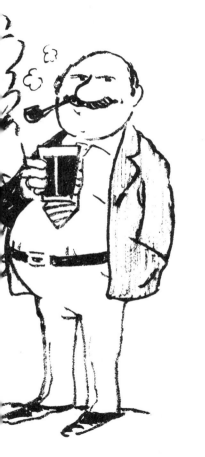

KEEP FIT WITH
DRINK

THE ALCOROBIC WAY
TO BUILD A
A BETTER BODY

Marcel Feigel
Illustrations by Brian Heaton

Practical guidance and technical advice by Dr. Brian Ferguson

FREDERICK MULLER

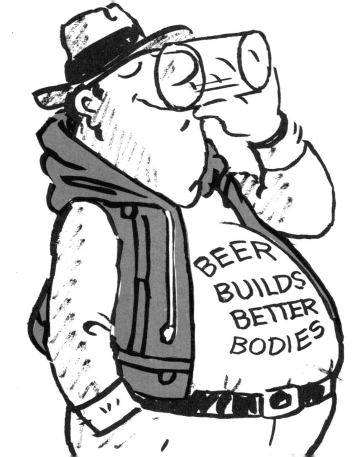

First published in Great Britain in 1984 by
Frederick Muller
Frederick Muller is an imprint of
Muller, Blond & White Limited,
55/57 Great Ormond Street, London
WC1N 3HZ

Feigel, Marcel
Keep fit with drink.
1. Drinking customs——Anecdotes, facetiae,
satire, etc.
I. Title
394.1'3'0207   GT2880

ISBN 0-584-11105-3

Printed and Bound in England
By R. J. Acford, Chichester, West Sussex

INTRODUCTION

Drinkers are like everybody else. They too would like to have lithe bodies and wear pastel sweatshirts and radiate good health (they may not admit it but they do).

But when it comes to exercise they're at a severe disadvantage. Because they simply haven't got the time. They're too busy doing other things — namely, drinking.

The trouble is that no one has taken the time to devise a fitness programme that would fit in with their lifestyle.

There are exercise programs for almost everybody else: for pregnant women and the handicapped, for the busy housewife and the man on the go, for the overweight and the undersexed.

But for drinkers? Nothing. Which is not only unfair but almost cruelly neglectful when you consider that there are so many. So we decided to do something about it.

If drinkers won't go to the gym, then there is only one thing to do: bring the gym to the drinkers. That's how alcorobics was born.

Here, finally, is just what the doctor ordered: a unique exercise system that can easily be practised in a pub, wine bar or at home. With a few exceptions (**see** *Corkscrews*) the exercises are very gentle so you won't have to worry about overextending yourself. In fact, you may have been doing many of the exercises for years, but just weren't aware of it.

The most important thing to realise is that these are exercises anybody can do. Even you. You don't need special clothes and if you miss a day there's no real sweat. Or should we say that if there is real sweat perhaps you should miss a day.

Which leaves only one thing left to do: open a bottle and get started.

SUGGESTED DRESS & POSTURE FOR ① PUBLIC HOUSE:

HAT LENDS DIGNITY

CORRECT DIRECTIONAL ROUTE KNOWLEDGE

STAIN RESISTANT SHIRT

*
WARM JACKET IN CASE OF HAVING TO STAY OUT ALL NIGHT

STRONG BELT BRACES OPTIONAL

GENERAL RELAXED ATTITUDE

A DOG (ANY BREED WILL DO) USEFUL FOR FINDING WAY HOME

FIRM TREAD

TROUSERS OF A LOOSE FIT ALLOWING FOR EXPANSION

* A STRONGLY DEVELOPED ABILITY TO AVERT WRATH.

SUGGESTED DRESS & POSTURE FOR ② WINE BARS

THOUGHTFUL HEAD POSITIONING

MEANINGFUL GAZE

SLIM PANTATELLA

LOTS OF HAIR TO FLING ABOUT

ABILITY TO STAY IN THIS POSITION FOR HOURS

SPRAY ON SUIT ADDS AUTHORITY IN CASE OF ARREST

IMMENSE CAPACITY FOR CONSUMING HOUSE WINE

ABILITY TO HOLD LOTS OF WHITE WINE & SODA WITHOUT VISITING THE GENTS TOO OFTEN.

LONG LEGS IF POSSIBLE

CONVERSATIONAL GAMBIT

MASCULINE MATURE STANCE (SEE ADS)

GOOD HEEL LOCK

POSITIONING
WRONG

POSITIONING RIGHT

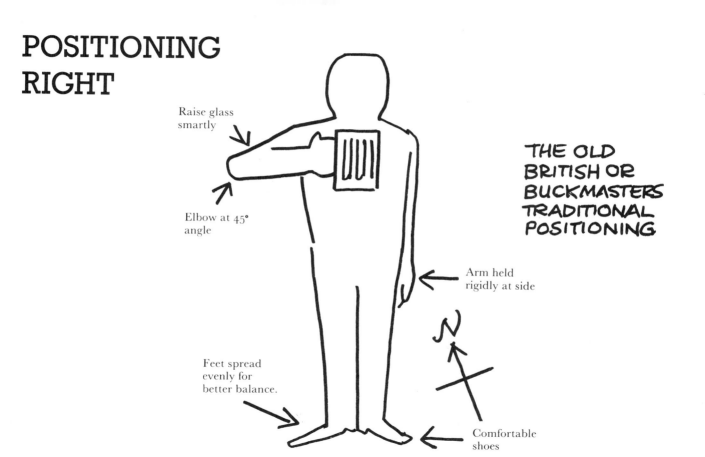

Raise glass smartly

Elbow at 45° angle

Feet spread evenly for better balance.

Arm held rigidly at side

Comfortable shoes

THE OLD BRITISH OR BUCKMASTERS TRADITIONAL POSITIONING

THE EXERCISES

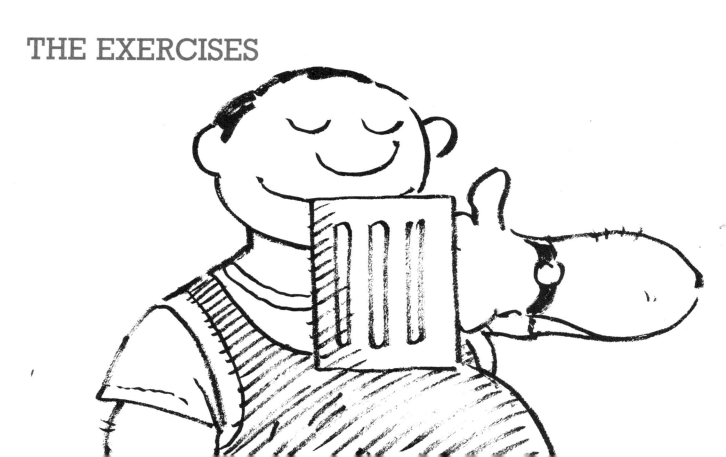

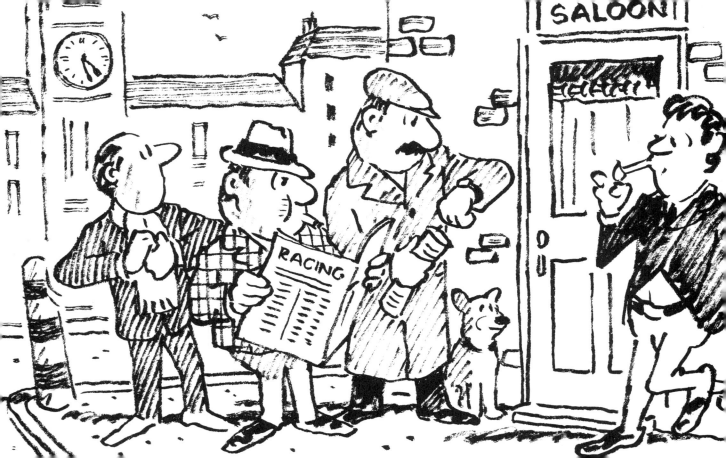

THE WARM UP

Limbering up is important before any kind of athletic activity and alcorobics is no exception. This is a good time to loosen up and get into the right mental state. Practise getting your hands into the starting position. Feel yourself leaning against the bar. Concentrate on getting the barman's attention. As before any major event, you'll probably experience some jitters but don't worry, they usually vanish as soon as the doors open.

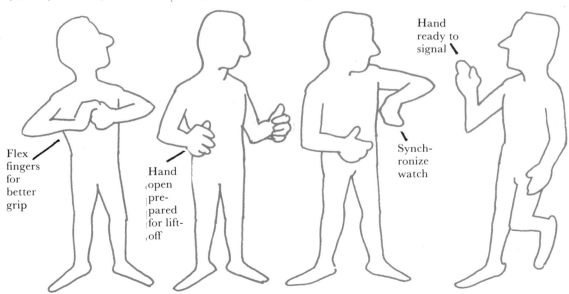

Flex fingers for better grip

Hand open prepared for lift-off

Hand ready to signal

Synchronize watch

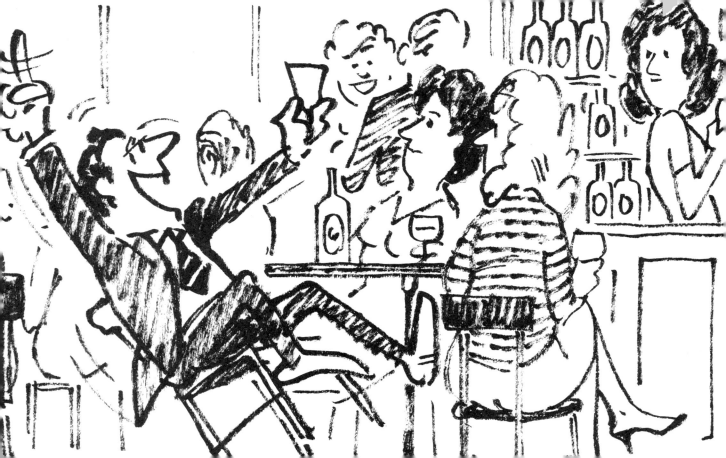

VERTICAL STRETCH

Raise your arm as high as you can, the higher the better — as if you were hailing a taxi. Then call out your order loud and clear: "Another jeroboam, please." Simple, isn't it! It's also fun. Best of all, the more you do it, the more you benefit. And so does everybody else.

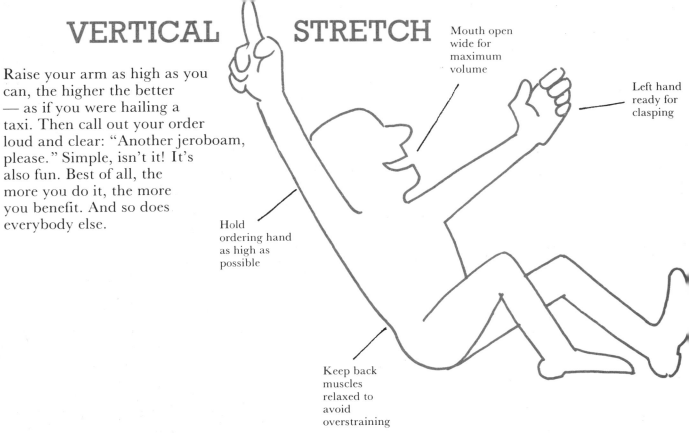

Mouth open wide for maximum volume

Left hand ready for clasping

Hold ordering hand as high as possible

Keep back muscles relaxed to avoid overstraining

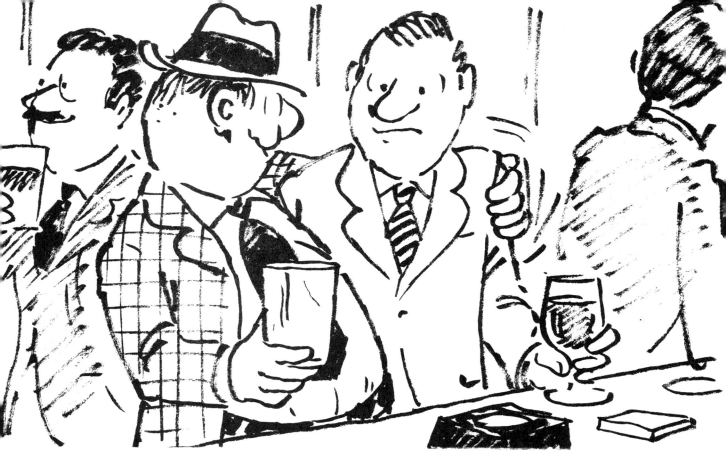

THE SQUEEZE

Pretend to suddenly recognize an old acquaintance just as he's about to buy a round. Quickly but casually stroll over and with your left hand give him a friendly hug.

Wait for a count of five, then with your right hand bring up an almost empty glass that will soon be re-filled free of charge, which is when the exercise ends. This is the simple squeeze. There is also an advanced version involving two glasses or even more, but that comes later.

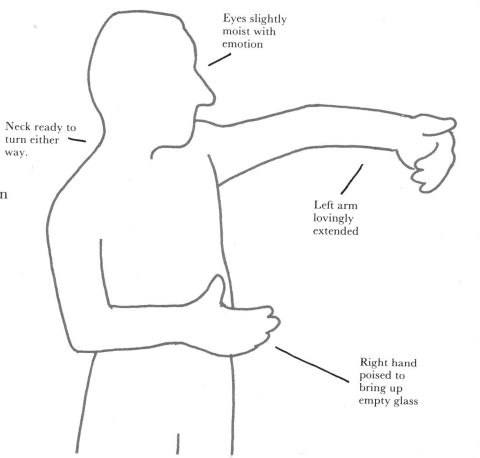

Eyes slightly moist with emotion

Neck ready to turn either way.

Left arm lovingly extended

Right hand poised to bring up empty glass

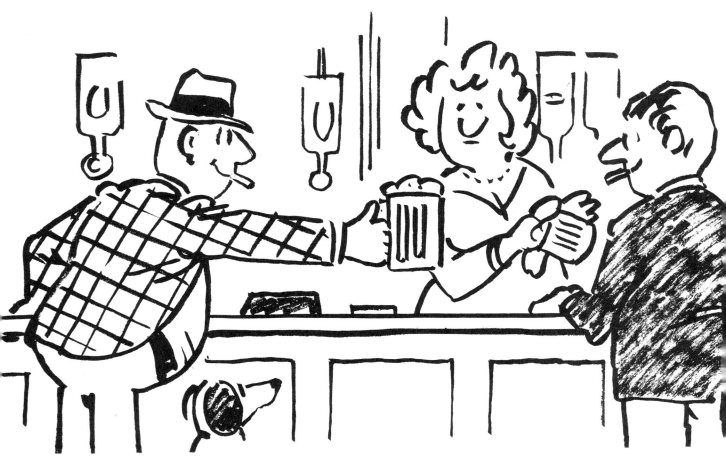

THE STRETCH

This is an exceptionally useful arm exercise that you can use again and again, especially in public places. The farther from the bar you are the better, because your arm has to stretch more. You'll find it particularly helpful when drinking with bores as by keeping them an arm or two arms' lengths away, you won't have to hear too much of what they are saying.

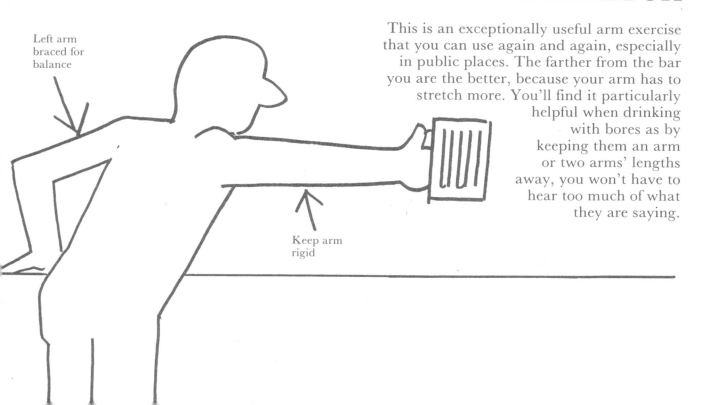

Left arm braced for balance

Keep arm rigid

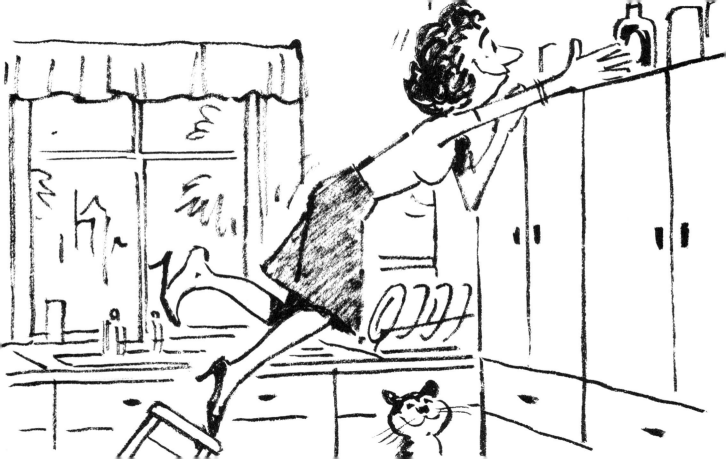

THE TIP TOE

Stand on tip toe and stretching as much as you can, reach for the bottle on top of the cupboard. Bring the bottle down slowly, have a swig and put it back up again keeping your right hand as steady as you can. Repeat the process four times, by which time you should be feeling a lot taller. Performed regularly, this exercise can also go a long way to relieve varicose veins and floppy discs.

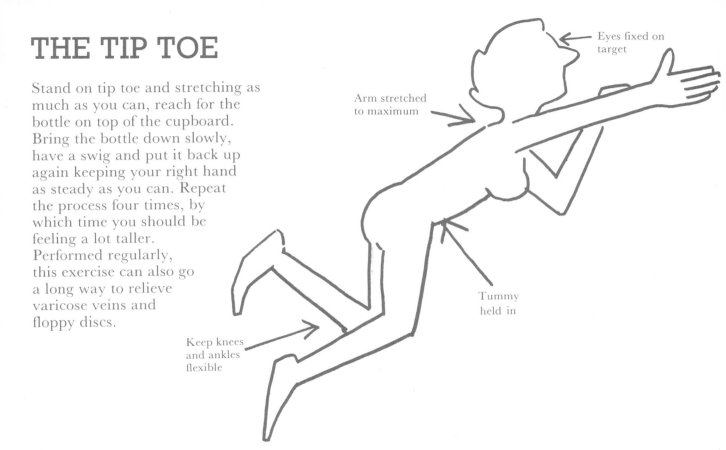

Eyes fixed on target

Arm stretched to maximum

Tummy held in

Keep knees and ankles flexible

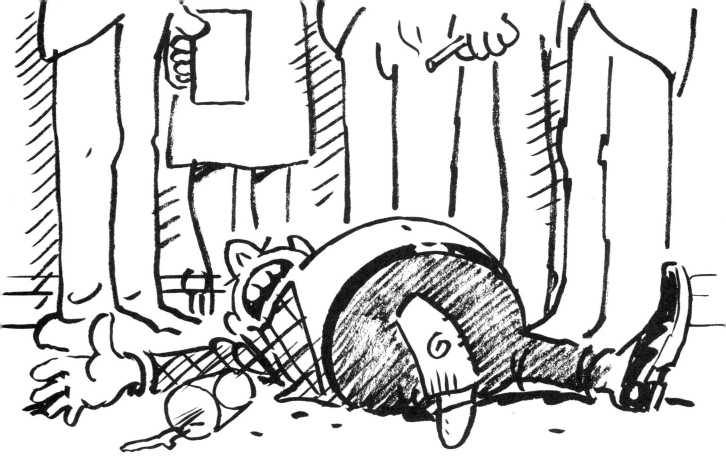

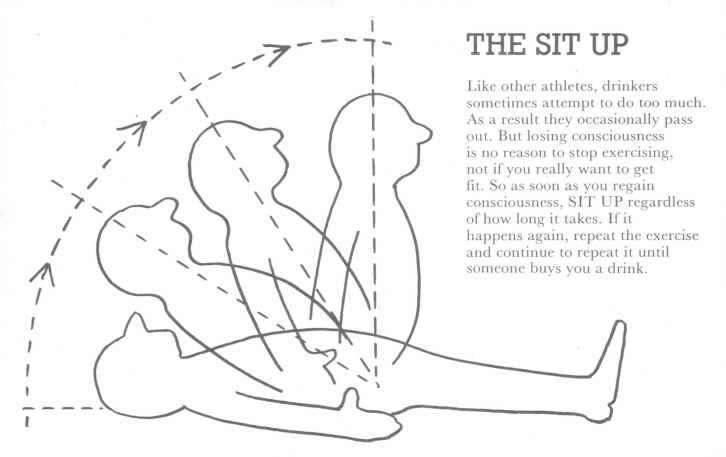

THE SIT UP

Like other athletes, drinkers
sometimes attempt to do too much.
As a result they occasionally pass
out. But losing consciousness
is no reason to stop exercising,
not if you really want to get
fit. So as soon as you regain
consciousness, SIT UP regardless
of how long it takes. If it
happens again, repeat the exercise
and continue to repeat it until
someone buys you a drink.

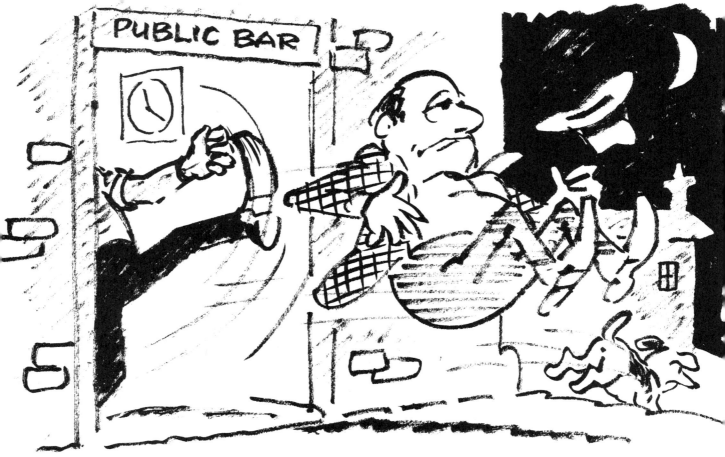

THE FALL

A classic self-defence exercise very similar to judo. You'll have to find an adversary — but for some reason pub landlords like to play this role.

To begin, let yourself go as limp as you can. This forces your adversary to provide most of the muscle power. As you're being thrown, make sure your legs are well in front of your body, and try to hit the pavement with your hands first, to break the fall.

One fall is usually enough. But if you feel like repeating the exercise, just go back inside, and order another drink.

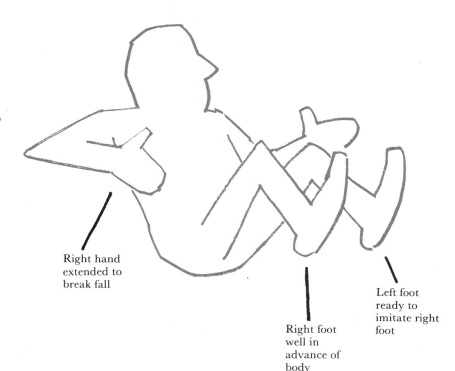

Right hand extended to break fall

Right foot well in advance of body

Left foot ready to imitate right foot

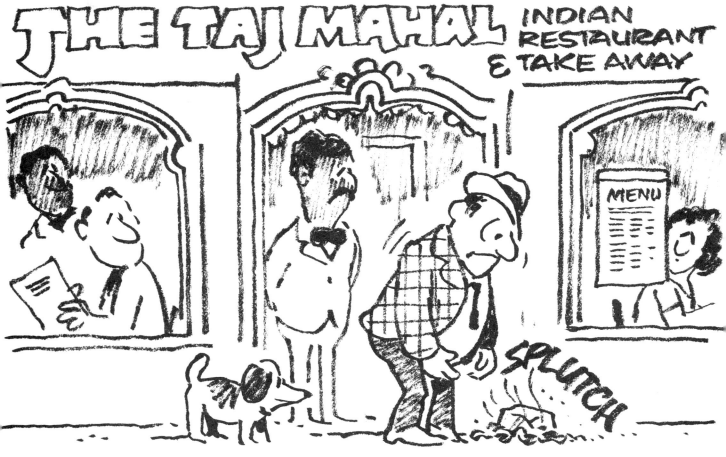

THE PICK-UP
RETRIEVING A CHICKEN VINDALOO

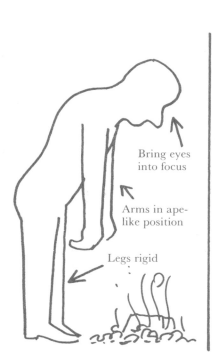

Bring eyes into focus

Arms in ape-like position

Legs rigid

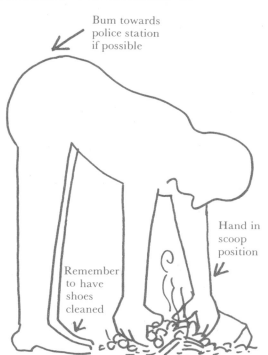

Bum towards police station if possible

Hand in scoop position

Remember to have shoes cleaned

This is a late night exercise that is particularly good for the back and spine and — if done properly — the stomach.

Stand as straight as you can (we know it's hard, but do your best) and slowly bend over until your hands are almost touching the ground. Then gracefully scrape the remnants of each dish back into its carton. If you can, try to breathe in time with the scooping.

When you've completed the pick-up, lick your fingers counter clockwise.

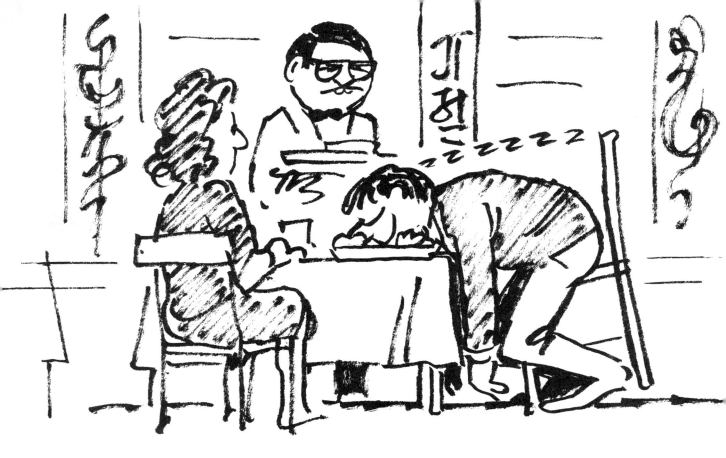

THE FORWARD LEAP

This is an excellent way to stop overeating. The key is establishing the right balance between how much you eat and drink. For each forkful of food you take in, drink one glass of wine. After ten forkfuls you should find your appetite starting to abate. Continue the exercise until your nose makes contact with the fettucini or creme caramel. Then take a short rest.

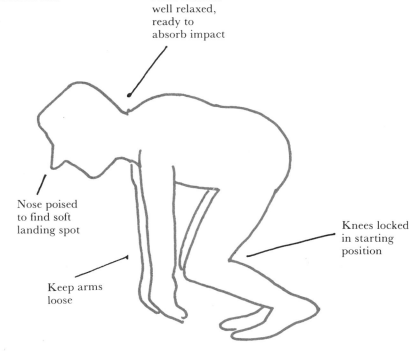

Neck muscles well relaxed, ready to absorb impact

Nose poised to find soft landing spot

Keep arms loose

Knees locked in starting position

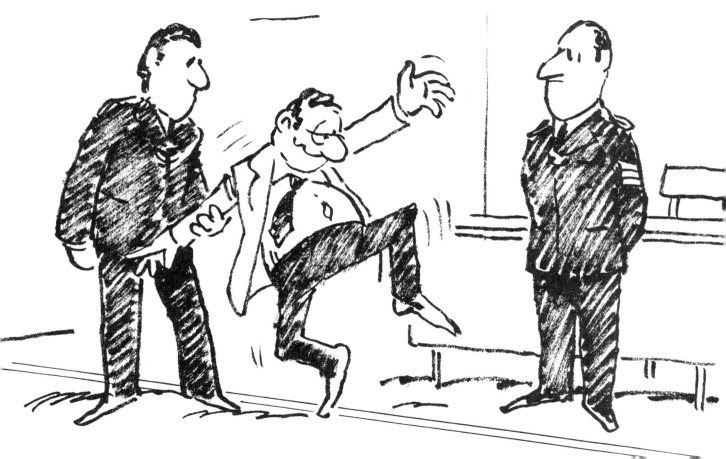

WALKING THE LINE

People who have difficulty walking a straight line also often find it hard to jitterbug. And for the same reason. It's so simple that it eludes them. So remember the old Chinese adage: "Think crooked and walk straight."

Once you've got the hang of it you'll be amazed how easy it can be. And you may be tempted to add little embellishments like clicking your heels or break-dancing. But it's best — for your sake and that of your loved ones — to keep it simple.

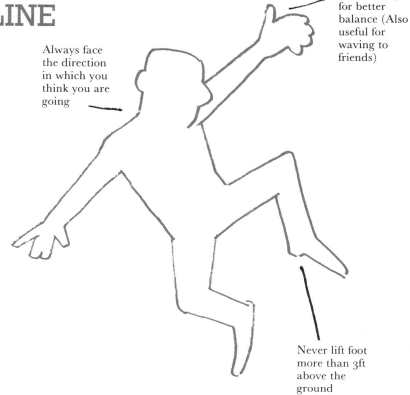

Always face the direction in which you think you are going

Lift arm high for better balance (Also useful for waving to friends)

Never lift foot more than 3ft above the ground

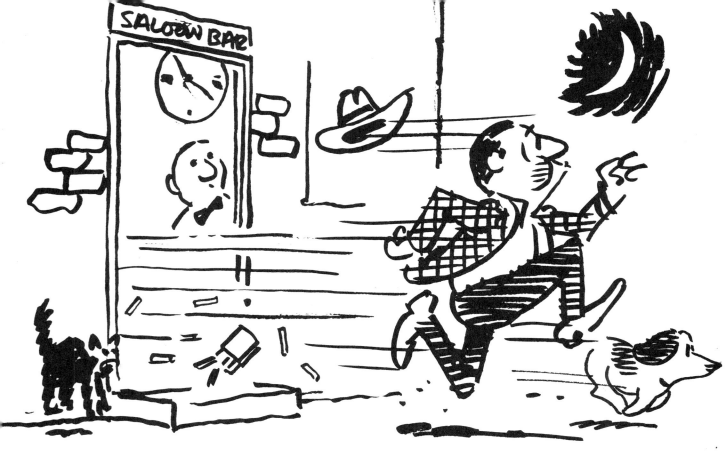

THE DASH
MISSING THE LAST BUS

As you're missing the last bus home, here are a few points to bear in mind. Keep your right arm as straight as you can and your left leg elevated at a 45° angle. This should add considerable spring to your step and get you in the mood for walking home. If done regularly this exercise should also improve your posture, make you look more alert — and do wonders for your street credibility.

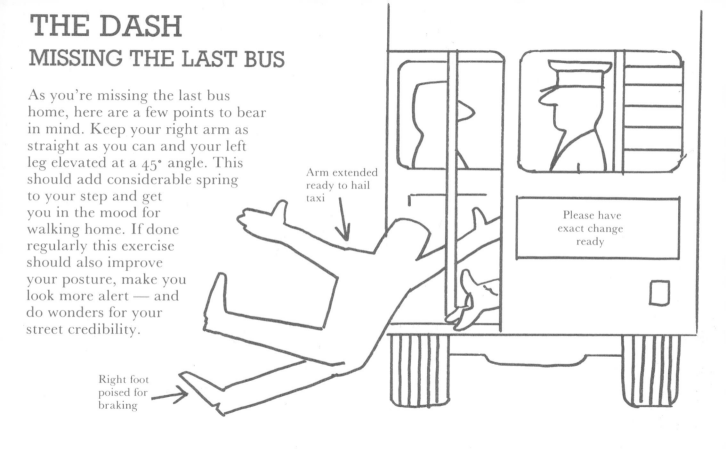

Arm extended ready to hail taxi

Please have exact change ready

Right foot poised for braking

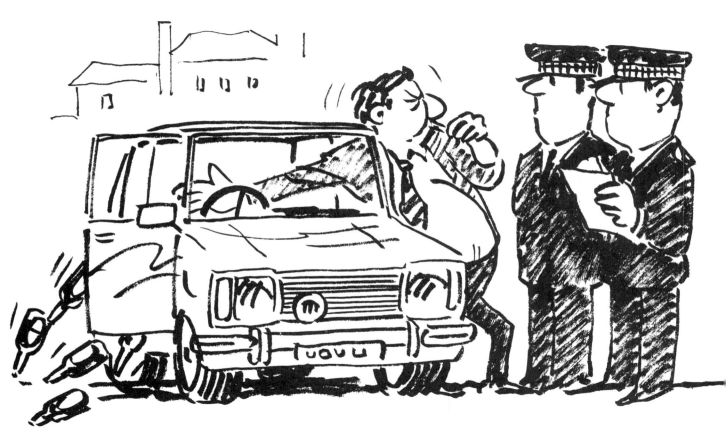

THE DEEP BREATH

This is a routine exercise whose sole function is to make sure that all the goodness from the alcohol is going straight into your bloodstream.

   As soon as you're handed the bag, blow into it as hard as you can. Don't rush. You've got plenty of time. If the bag turns a vivid green, then you've passed with flying colours. If not, then drive to the nearest pub and have a few more.

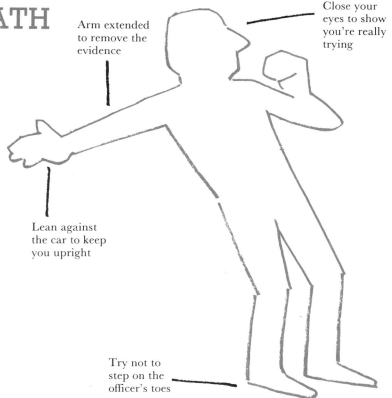

Arm extended to remove the evidence

Close your eyes to show you're really trying

Lean against the car to keep you upright

Try not to step on the officer's toes

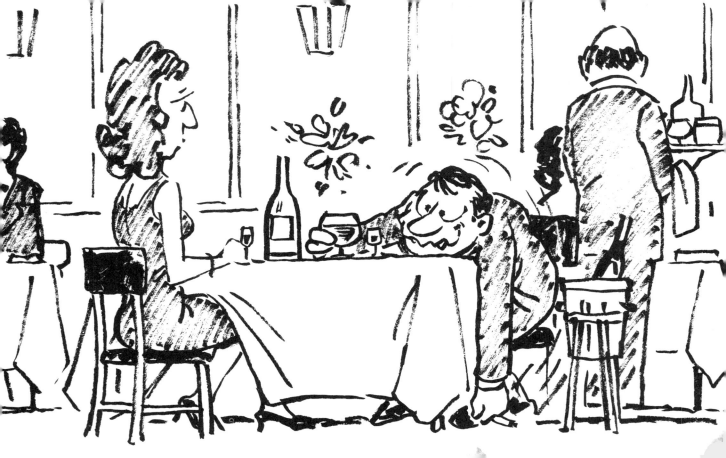

THE ROLL

This is an after dinner exercise designed to ease the digestive process. First, place your face gently on the table. Then slowly but steadily follow your body's natural gravitational pull which, you'll observe, follows a centripetal path. Try to maintain an even arc-like descent which should lead to a soft touchdown. Very good for the lower lumbar region.

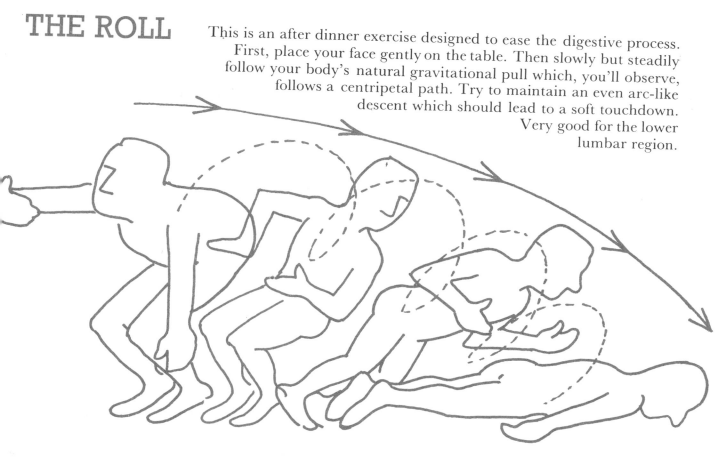

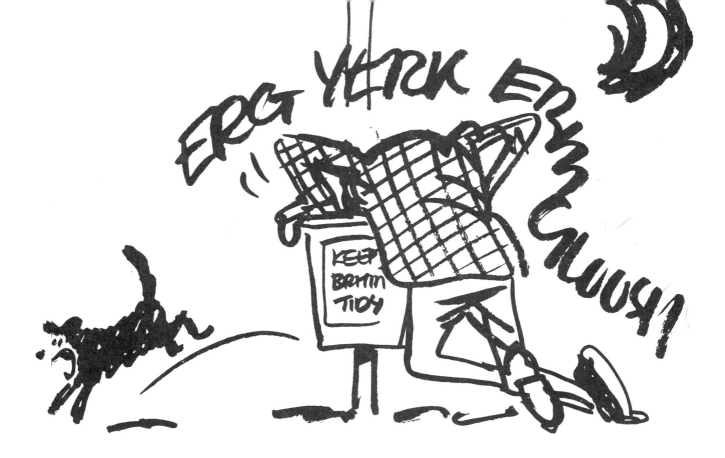

THE HEAVE

One of the most important exercises you can do.
In fact, many experienced exercisers make it part
of their daily routine. It has a multitude of
benefits but is particularly beneficial to the
abdominal muscles, especially the
involuntary muscles which work very
hard without knowing it. Many people
find it difficult at first but it
gets easier as you go along.
It's good for skin tone, relaxes the
mind, eliminates dandruff and makes
your whole body feel a lot lighter.
So it's not surprising that it's so
popular. It's also one of the few
exercises you don't have
to repeat. Chances are
it will repeat itself.

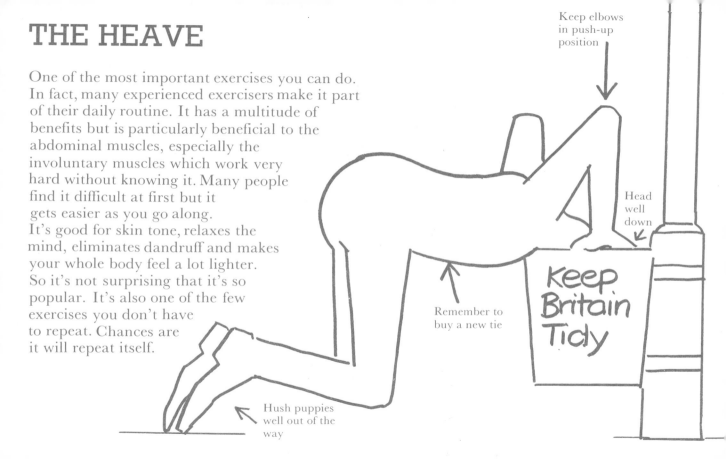

Keep elbows
in push-up
position

Head
well
down

Remember to
buy a new tie

Keep
Britain
Tidy

Hush puppies
well out of the
way

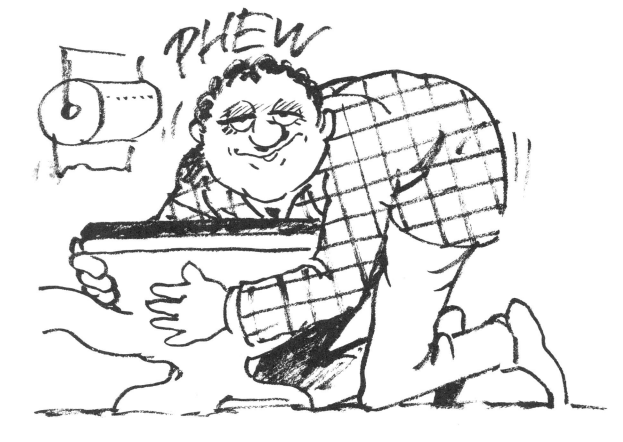

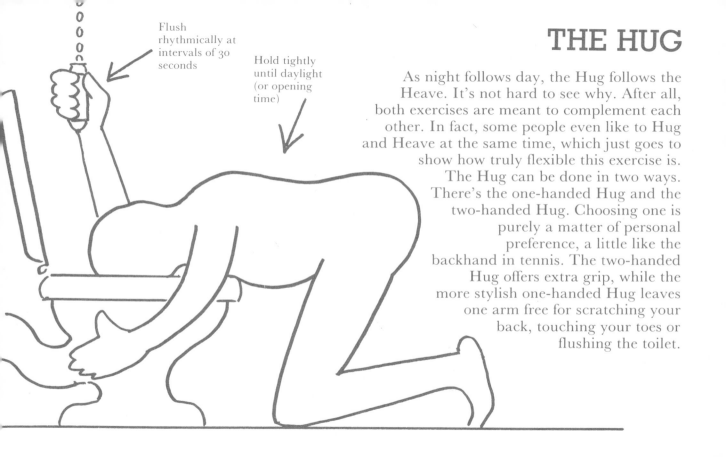

Flush rhythmically at intervals of 30 seconds

Hold tightly until daylight (or opening time)

THE HUG

As night follows day, the Hug follows the Heave. It's not hard to see why. After all, both exercises are meant to complement each other. In fact, some people even like to Hug and Heave at the same time, which just goes to show how truly flexible this exercise is. The Hug can be done in two ways. There's the one-handed Hug and the two-handed Hug. Choosing one is purely a matter of personal preference, a little like the backhand in tennis. The two-handed Hug offers extra grip, while the more stylish one-handed Hug leaves one arm free for scratching your back, touching your toes or flushing the toilet.

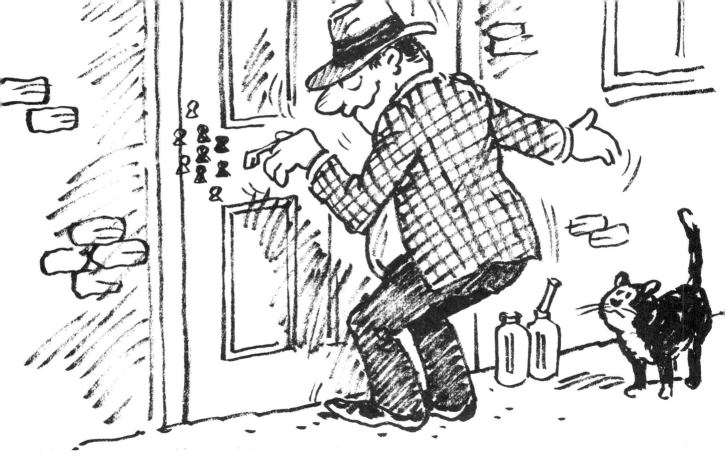

THE INSERTION

This is a very demanding exercise so don't be surprised if you don't get it at the first try. Very few people do. It calls for superb reflexes, split second timing, and the concentration of a test pilot. What makes it even more difficult is that, as we all know, keyholes tend to move. But be persistent. Eventually you'll get there. In the meantime, remember, even if you miss, extricating your nose from the letterbox can also be a constructive exercise.

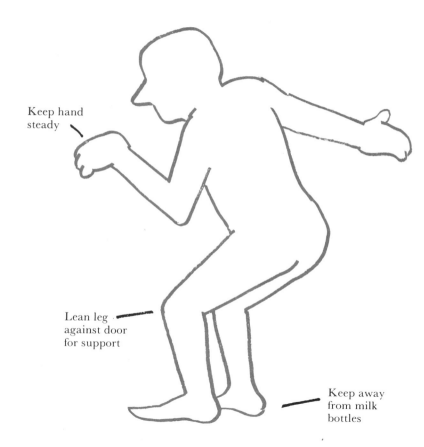

Keep hand steady

Lean leg against door for support

Keep away from milk bottles

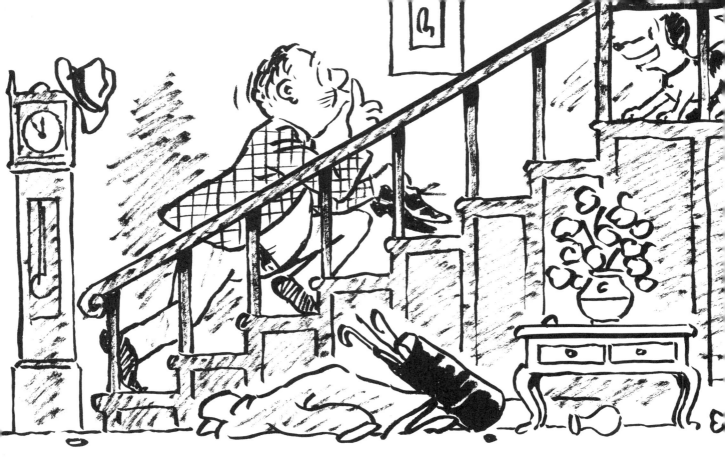

THE CLIMB

A very delicate and very important exercise, perhaps the most important exercise in this book. Because it could play a large part in your future well-being. And if you do it wrong, you may not get another chance. The crucial factor with this exercise is that it must be performed in SILENCE. So try not to drop your shoes. Remember to carry a bone for the dog. And above all, maintain your balance, because falling down the stairs could be fatal.

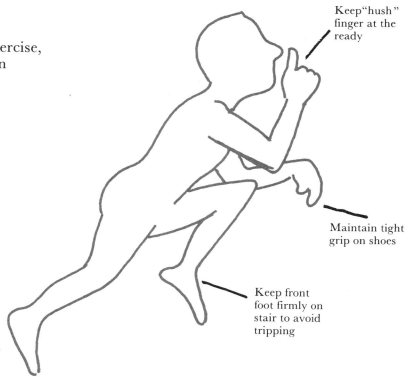

Keep "hush" finger at the ready

Maintain tight grip on shoes

Keep front foot firmly on stair to avoid tripping

Back foot ready to retreat

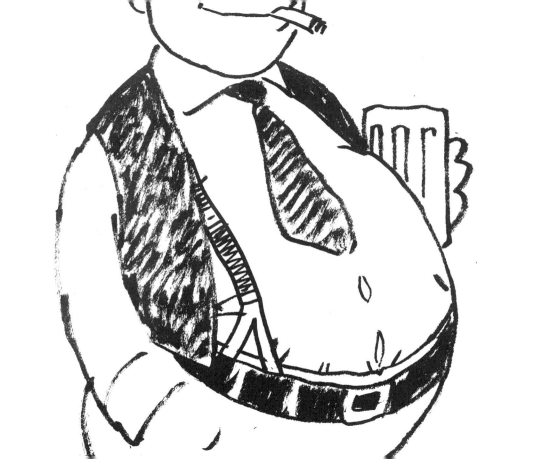

STOMACH EXERCISES

You can tell a lot about people from the places they hang out. The original gravity of a person's stomach can also be revealing. But too many people make the mistake of thinking that the only way of doing away with the flab is by doing away with the drinks. Which is a little like saying that the only way to silence a mother-in-law is by getting divorced.

Fortunately, the alcorobic attitude is far more enlightened. We realise that this is an area that often needs special attention. That's why we have come up with our own unique series of exercises that gently coax your tummy into flatness without - as happens too often - resorting to intimidation or violence.

The best way to benefit from this regime is to first find your stomach type, then choose the exercises that suit you best.

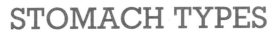

STOMACH TYPES

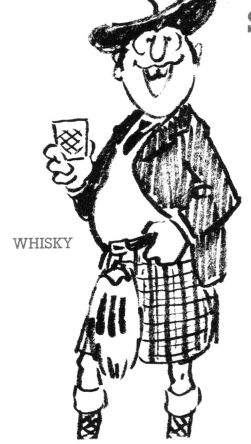

WHISKY

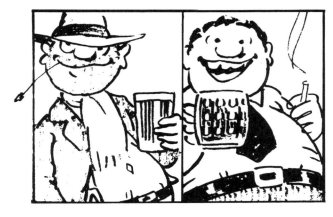

SCRUMPY   REAL ALE

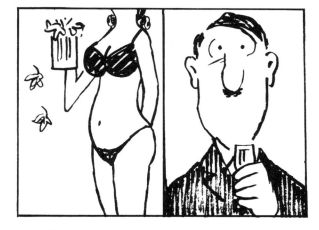

PIMM'S No 1   SCHNAPPS

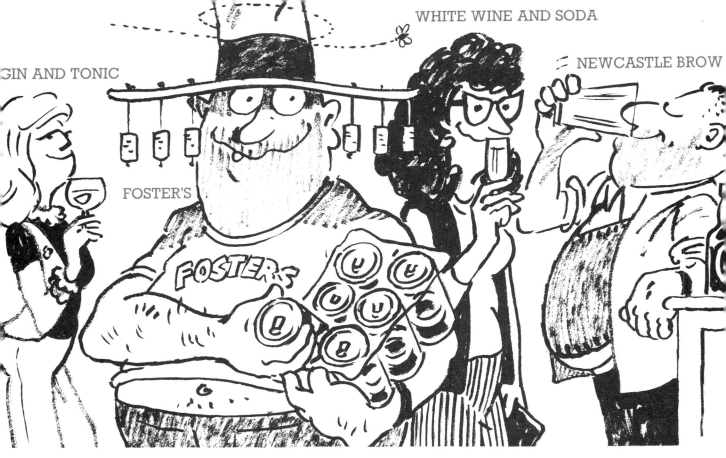

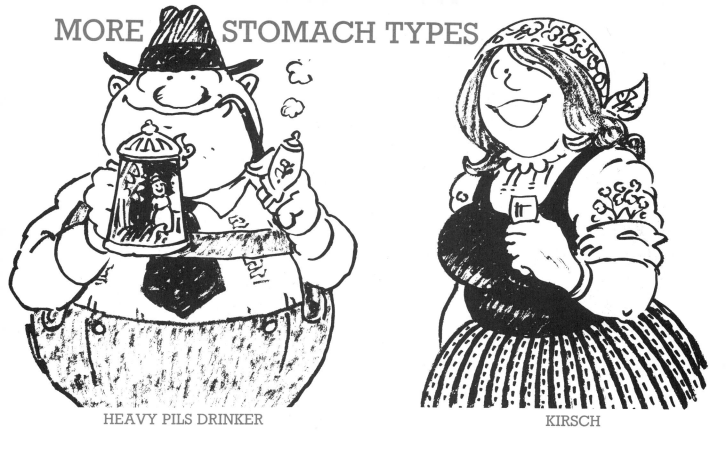

MORE STOMACH TYPES

HEAVY PILS DRINKER   KIRSCH

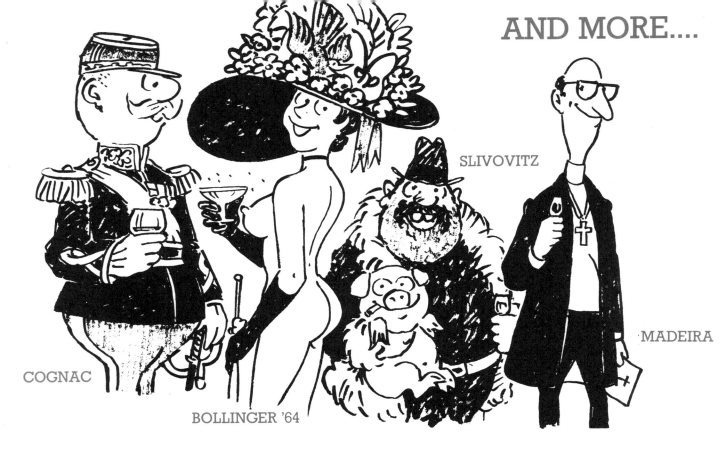

AND MORE....

COGNAC

BOLLINGER '64

SLIVOVITZ

MADEIRA

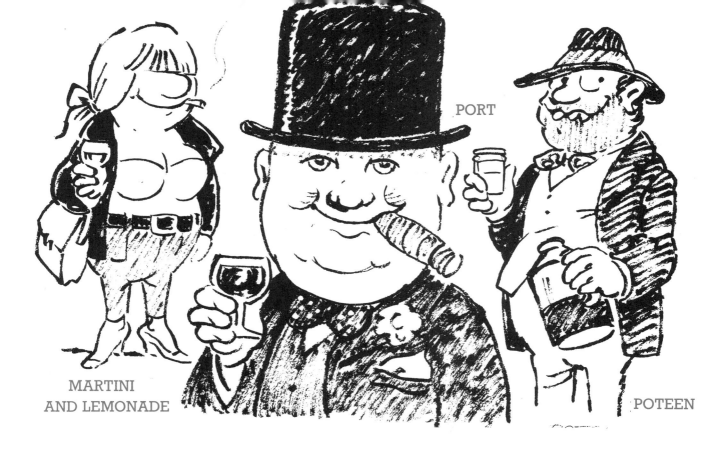

STOMACH EXERCISES

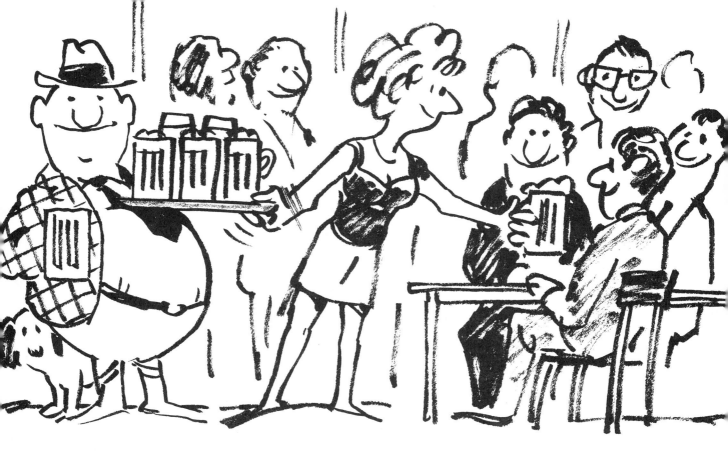

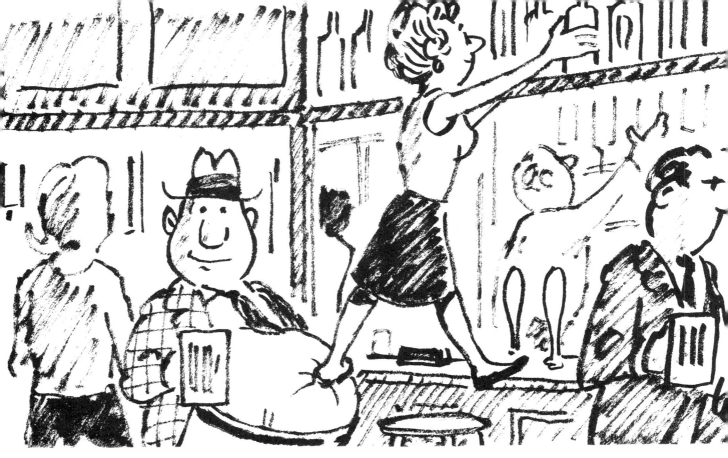

MORE STOMACH EXERCISES

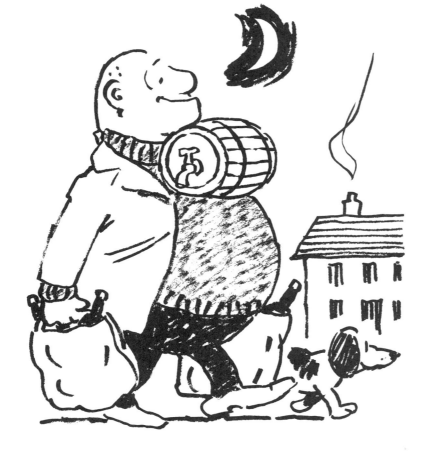

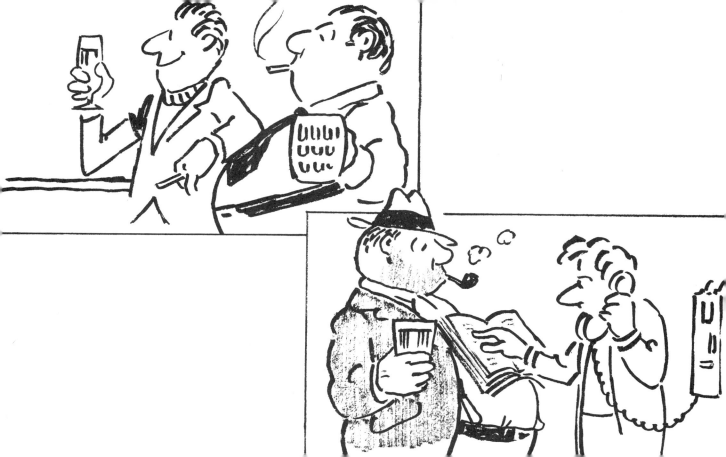

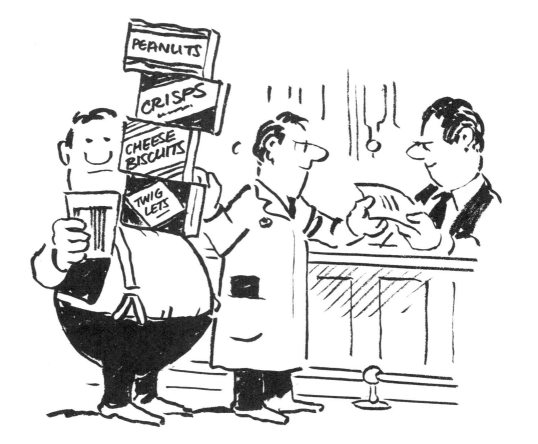

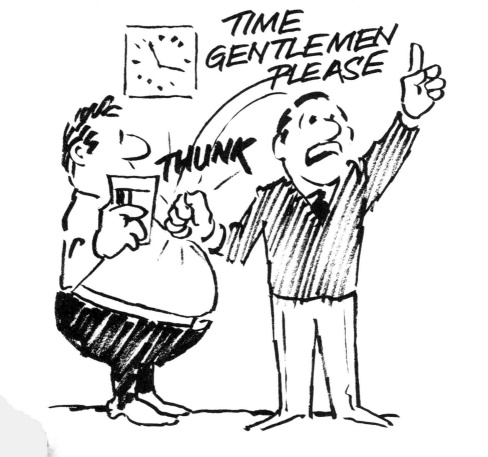

AND MORE....

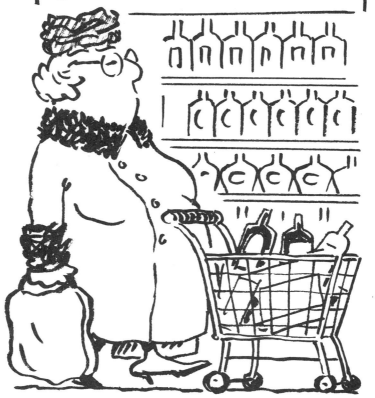

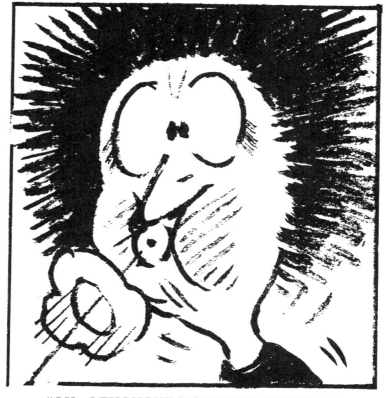

"OH - I THOUGHT YOU LIKED TEQUILA"

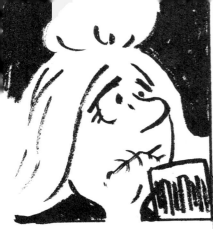

THE FIRST HALF EVER

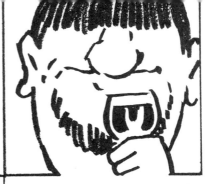

BEAUJOLAIS NOUVEAU

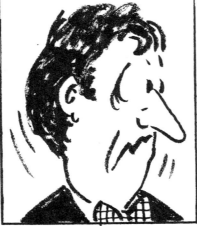

ON SEEING A CREDITOR

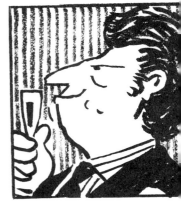

CONNOISSEUR

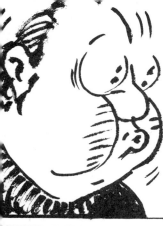

AFTER A PINT IN ONE

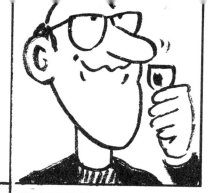

"SLIGHTLY DRY I THINK"

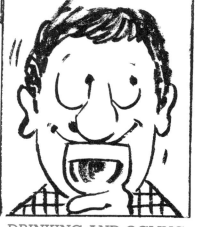

DRINKING AND OGLING

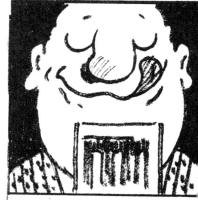

SATISFACTION
AT THE FIRST SIP

FACIAL EXERCISES

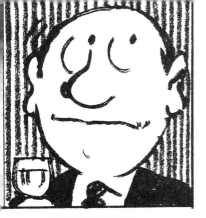

"VERY NICE
ELDERBERRY"

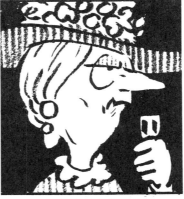

SHERRY TASTING

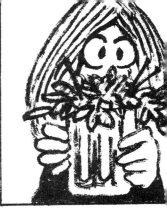

PIMMS No.1

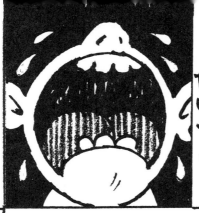

BAD BUDGET NEWS

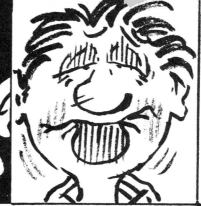

MORNING
TONGUE EXERCISE

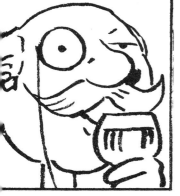

ON BEING BOUGHT
A DRINK

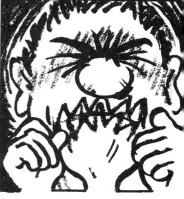

HAVING DROPPED
THE WHOLE TRAY

THE ALCOROBIC WAY....

The key to exercise is repetition.

The more you repeat a movement the more benefit you derive from it. This applies to opening wine just as much as it does to pumping iron, doing press ups or hitting golf balls.

The more bottles you open, the fitter you'll be. But don't try to do too much too soon: start with a case and gradually work your way up.

You should, of course, be drinking as you're opening. Otherwise you won't be getting the full alcorobic benefit.

Don't forget that the purpose of alcorobics (like aerobics) is to increase your heart beat for short bursts. So try measuring your pulse after every three bottles you consume. If your pulse hasn't doubled after the first nine bottles then switch to champagne.

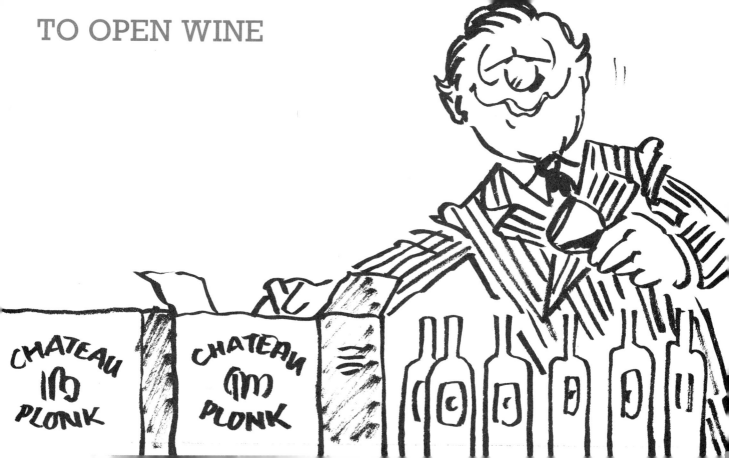

TO OPEN WINE

CORKSCREWS

Athletes are only as good as their equipment. Racing drivers have their Formula Ones, golfers have their clubs, tennis players their racquets.

You have your corkscrew.

But finding the right corkscrew is very important. Forget gadgets. Remember, half the fun of opening wine is the strain. That's why an old fashioned model is the best.

To get the maximum benefit from your corkscrew try to find a wine with a cork that offers some resistance. For this, basic Spanish reds are highly recommended, preferably those that cost under £1.50 a bottle. You'll be amazed at the difference it makes to the muscles in your arms - and in your forehead.

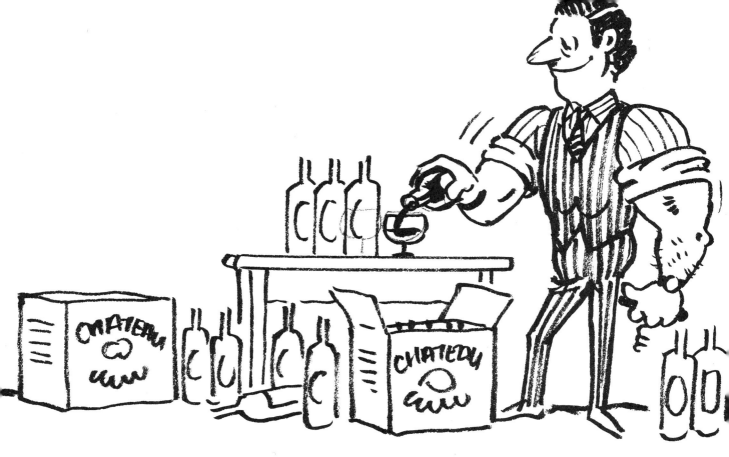

CORKSCREWS AND OTHER OPENING METHODS

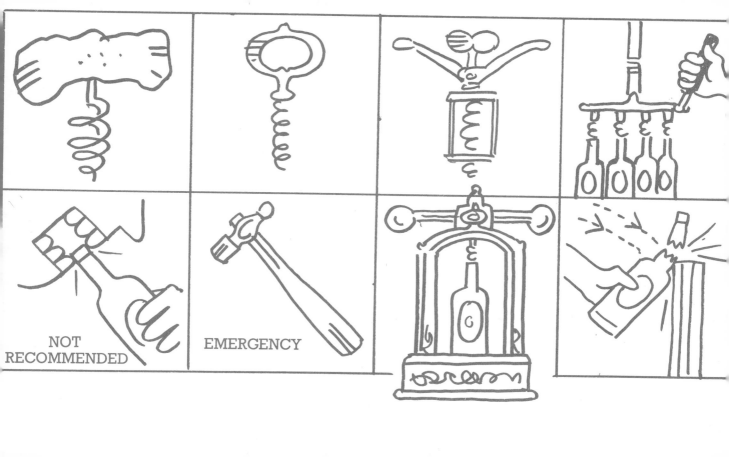

NOT
RECOMMENDED

EMERGENCY

AT THE SAUNA

We all know that saunas are good for you. But let's face it, they're pretty boring. However, as some of our Nordic friends have discovered, there is a way of making saunas a lot more interesting. It's simply a question of how you go about it. They've learned that a little alcohol artfully ladled over the coals can do more than water ever can.

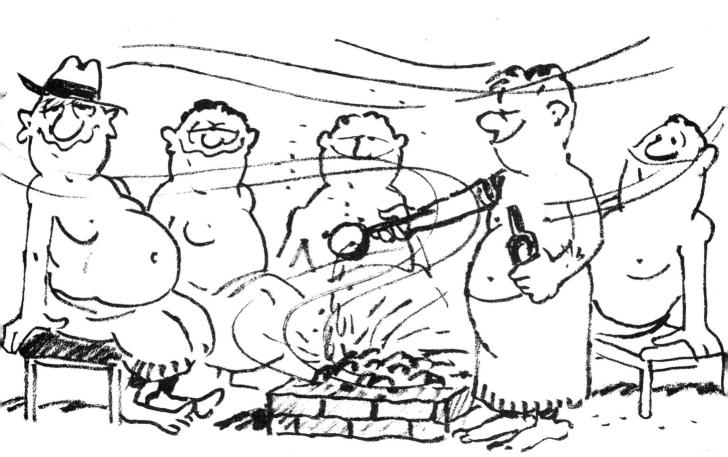

SAUNA ALCOHOL CHART

MORNING	NOON
Bull's Blood	Pernod
Southern Comfort	Muscadet
Sherry	Rioja
Liebfraumilch	Sake
Tequila	Whisky Mac (for wet weather)
Buck's Fizz	Guinness (the perfect alcorobic lunch)
Schlitz (great with corn-flakes but OK in the sauna too)	Chianti (very pleasant and the straw burns well)
Watney's Red Barrel (but only in Spain)	Beaujolais Nouveau (but never after Nov. 14)
Elderberry Wine	

WHAT TO POUR OVER THE COALS

NIGHT	WEE HOURS
Claret (for Boys)	Slivovitz
Port (for Men)	Old Spice
Brandy (for Heroes)	Communion Wine
Champagne (for Lovers)	Dr. Collis Browne's (but read the leaflet first)
Corrida (for Cheapskates)	Tesco's Own Lambrusco
Jameson's Irish Whiskey	Babycham (but there must be at least one girl under 16 present)
Bailey's (for family groups only)	Ouzo (remember that dusty bottle you brought back from Corfu?)
Jack Daniels (but only with appropriate music)	Methylated Spirits (but have extra coal ready)
Absinthe	

NOTE Under no circumstances use Foster's *even* if Australia has just won the test. The same goes for cider and scrumpy.

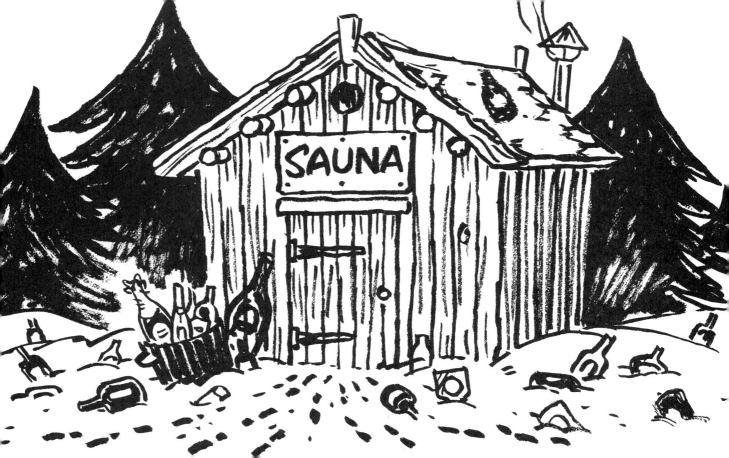

APRÈS SAUNA

After a good sauna most people feel very relaxed. After an alcorobic sauna you'll find you're so relaxed you probably won't even feel like going out.

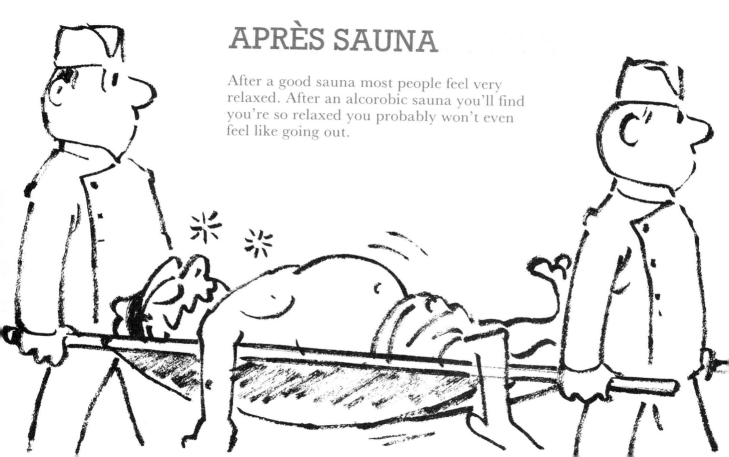

MENTAL EXERCISES

One of the best things about alcorobics is that it's not just limited to physical exercise. Like yoga, it aims to develop the whole person.

That's why we're devoting a whole section to mental exercises.

Mental exercises are important for clearing and strengthening the mind. It's especially important to perform them in the morning, usually as soon as you wake up.

A good way to start is by asking yourself a few questions while you're still lying in bed.

Some useful questions are:
1) Who am I?
2) Where am I?
3) Where did I leave my raincoat?

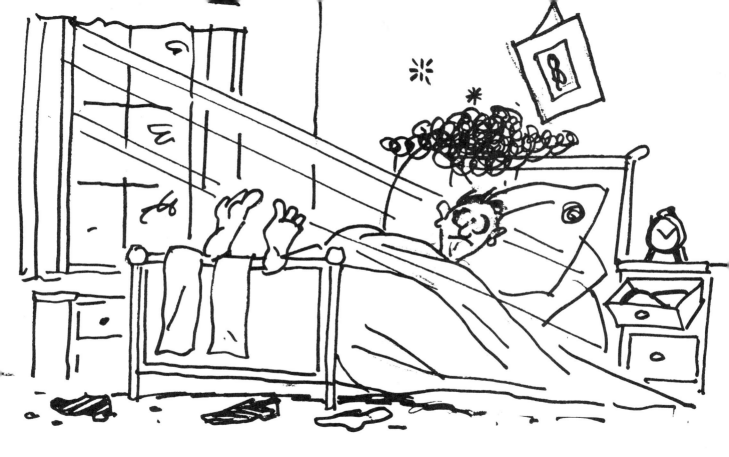

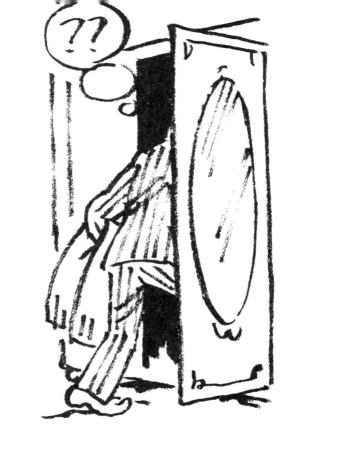

MENTAL EXERCISES

Now, mustering all of your strength, get out of bed and find your way to the bathroom. Don't be afraid to use your hands. Remember, alcorobics involves the complete totality of the individual and that includes developing your tactile sense.

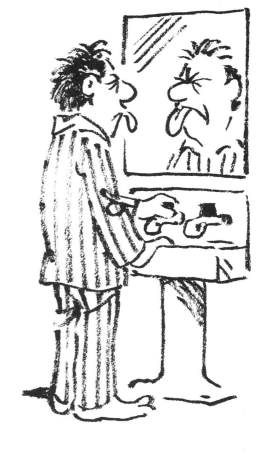

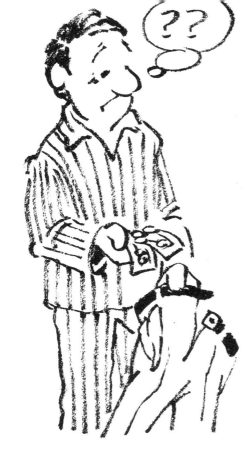

As soon as you return walk over to where you think you left your trousers. Don't panic if you can't find them immediately. They must be somewhere in the room, musn't they?

When you've found them, reach into your right hand pocket and see how much money is inside. You may have to reach inside several times because pound notes tend to crumple after midnight. Also because you're likely to run into a baffling assortment of items ranging from old cleaning tickets to ladies' undergarments. Disregard these for the moment, and just concentrate on the money. This should be easy enough since there won't be very much - usually around £1.89. At this point some people go into a frenzy desperately searching for that tenner that they knew was there. Don't bother. You won't find it.

Now with your worldly wealth clutched firmly in your shaking hand, calmly try to remember how much you started with last night and how you spent it. This is an exercise that could take all day. At first the answer may come as a blur. But eventually the whole picture will unfold with a vividness that will startle you, which is a testament to the force and clarity your mind can achieve.

This is just one example of mental alcorobics in action. With a little practise you can find literally hundreds more. Thanks to the magic of alcorobics you'll find that even the most menial task can tax the mind. And trying to remember the simplest fact - like where you parked your car - can be a mentally stimulating experience. Which all adds immeasurable mental enrichment to your daily life, not to mention weekends.

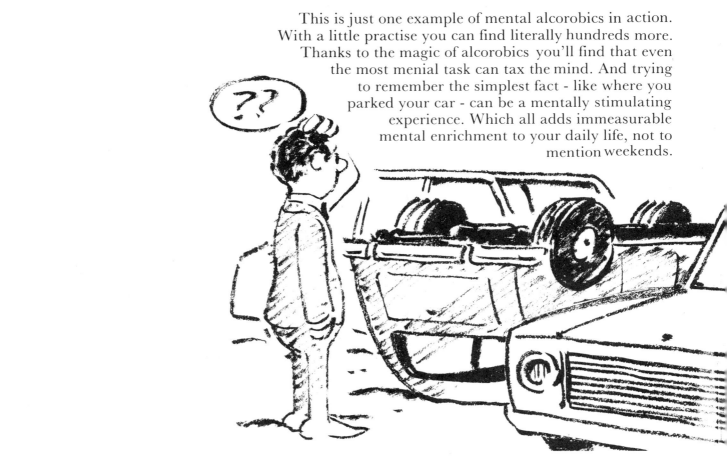

AILMENTS AND THEIR REMEDIES

Any intensive programme of exercise is bound to result occasionally in injuries. Alcorobics is no exception. That's why we have devised a special range of alcopathic remedies that are particularly effective at providing fast relief.

For minor injuries we recommend that you go to your local. They may not sell band-aids, but they do know how to get you plastered.

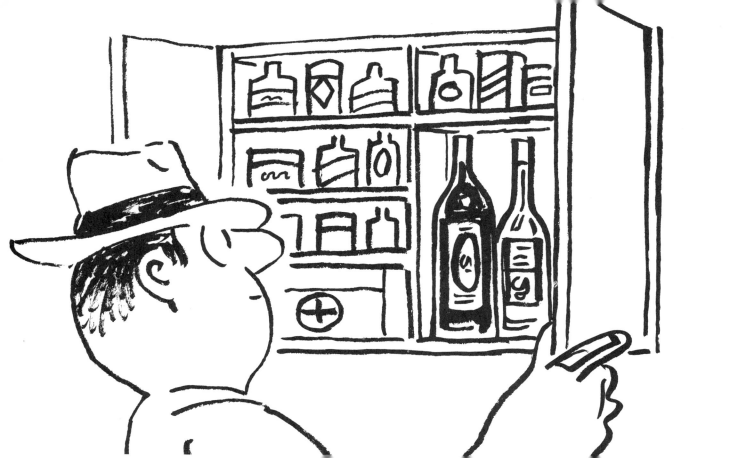

AILMENTS AND THEIR REMEDIES

AILMENT	ALCOPATHIC REMEDY
Broken bones	Singapore Sling
Impotence	Bull's Blood
Athlete's foot	Rusty Nail
Throbbing pain in the neck form not having registered for value added tax.	VAT 69
Nervous disorders due to legal troubles	Advocaat
Headaches	Two Pils before going to bed

AILMENT	ALCOPATHIC REMEDY
Depression	Tequila Sunrise
Lack of sparkle	Magnum Force
Numbness caused by too much exercise with heavy metal	Harvey Wallbanger
Inability to interact with others	Sancerre
Bunyons	Johnny Walker
Inertia caused by reading too much high brow literature	Lowenbrau
Gastric upset caused by eating too many hot curries	Vin de Loo

THE BRANDY ALEXANDER

One of the most dramatic advances in fitness therapy is the Alexander Technique which resolves physical and neurological problems through restructuring your posture.

We've developed a technique of our own which works on the same principle but with far less effort, and considerably more fun.

The basic technique is remarkably simple. Shortly after waking, quickly down three Brandy Alexanders. This should make you feel a lot taller. Continue the exercise until you reach your desired height.

Don't worry about becoming too tall as this exercise comes with its own built-in safety measure. As soon as you exceed your optimum height, a mental trigger goes off and quickly brings you back down to earth.

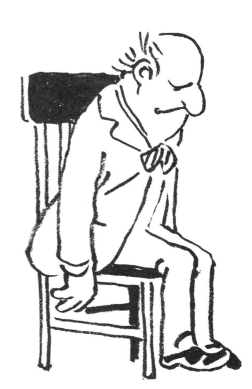

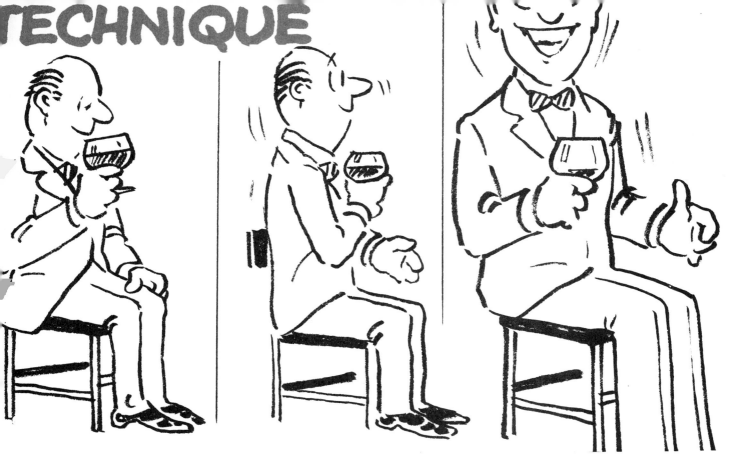

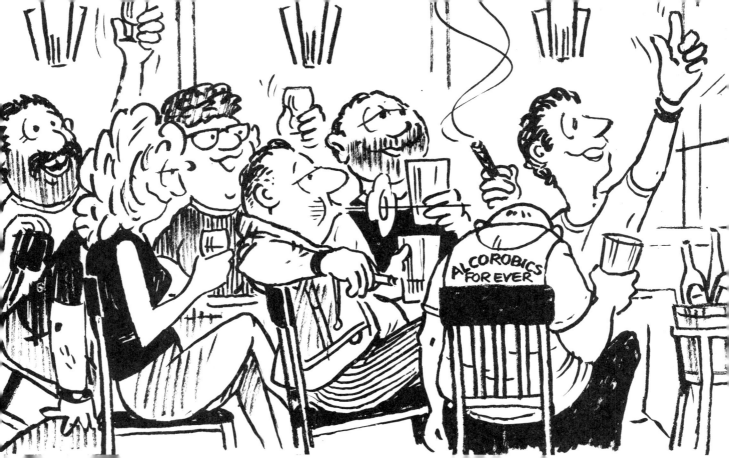

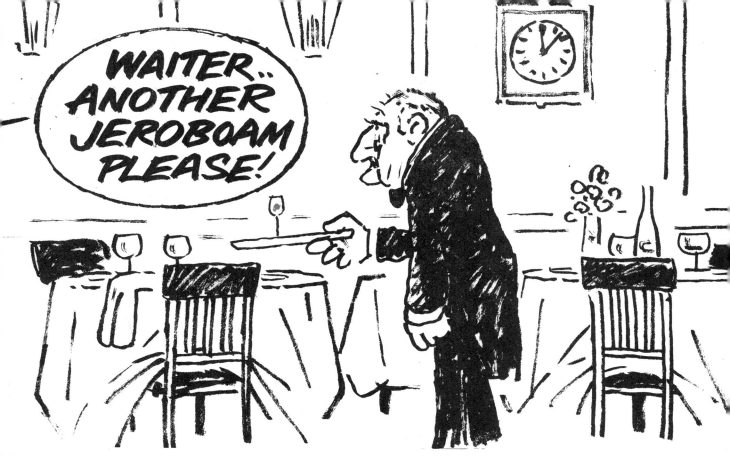

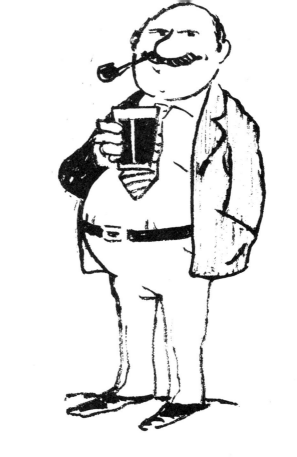